D0776894

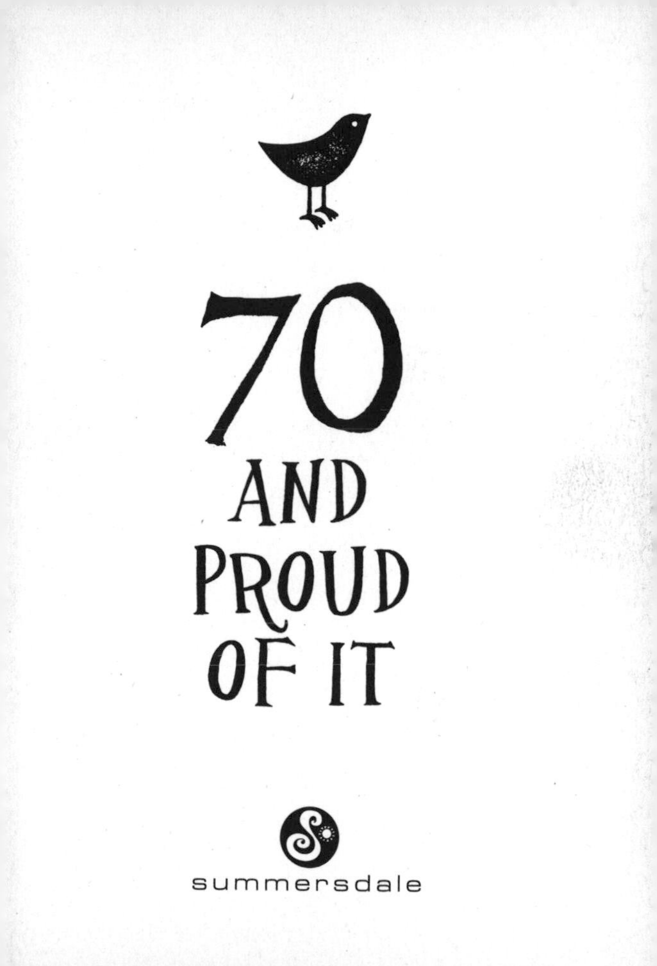
70
AND
PROUD
OF IT
summersdale

70 AND PROUD OF IT

With text contributed by Vicky Edwards

Summersdale Publishers Ltd
46 West Street
Chichester
West Sussex
PO19 1RP
UK

www.summersdale.com

Printed and bound in the Czech Republic

ISBN: 978-1-84953-565-6

TO...

FROM.......................................

CONTENTS

ANOTHER YEAR OLDER

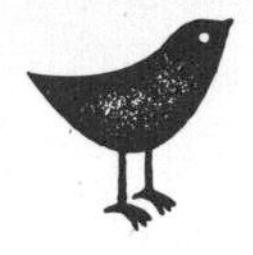

BEING 70 IS NO DIFFERENT FROM BEING 69. IT'S A ROUND NUMBER, AND THERE'S SOMETHING ABOUT ROUNDNESS THAT HAS ALWAYS APPEALED.

Elizabeth Taylor

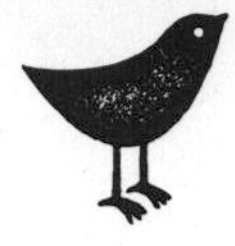

TO BE 70 YEARS YOUNG IS SOMETIMES FAR MORE CHEERFUL AND HOPEFUL THAN TO BE 40 YEARS OLD.

Oliver Wendell Holmes Jr

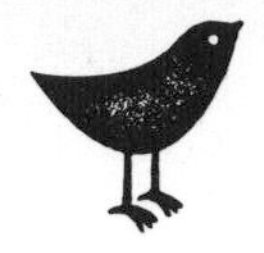

OUR WRINKLES ARE OUR MEDALS OF THE PASSAGE OF LIFE. THEY ARE WHAT WE HAVE BEEN THROUGH AND WHO WE WANT TO BE.

Lauren Hutton

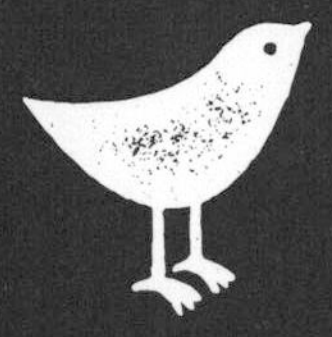

THERE WAS A STAR DANCED, AND UNDER THAT WAS I BORN.

William Shakespeare

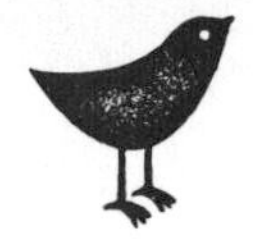

BIRTHDAYS ARE GOOD FOR YOU. STATISTICS SHOW THAT THE PEOPLE WHO HAVE THE MOST LIVE THE LONGEST.

Larry Lorenzoni

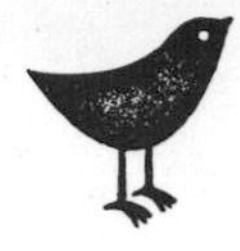

A BIRTHDAY IS JUST THE FIRST DAY OF ANOTHER 365-DAY JOURNEY AROUND THE SUN. ENJOY THE TRIP.

Anonymous

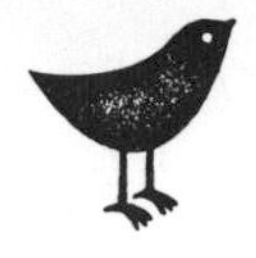

OUR BIRTHDAYS ARE FEATHERS IN THE BROAD WING OF TIME.

Jean Paul

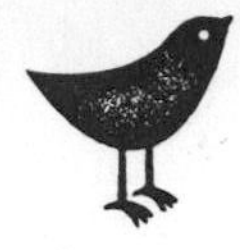

EVENTUALLY YOU WILL REACH A POINT IN LIFE WHEN YOU STOP LYING ABOUT YOUR AGE AND START BRAGGING ABOUT IT.

Will Rogers

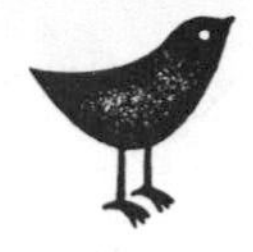

WHATEVER WITH THE
PAST HAS GONE,
THE BEST IS ALWAYS
YET TO COME.

Lucy Larcom

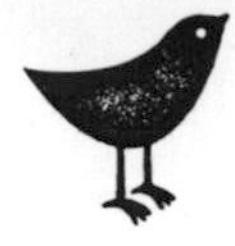

EACH TEN YEARS OF
A MAN'S LIFE HAS ITS
OWN FORTUNES, ITS OWN
HOPES, ITS OWN DESIRES.

Johann Wolfgang von Goethe

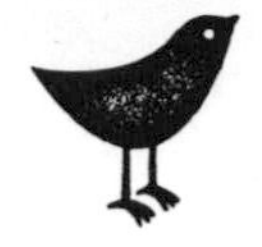

PLEAS'D TO LOOK FORWARD, PLEAS'D TO LOOK BEHIND, AND COUNT EACH BIRTHDAY WITH A GRATEFUL MIND.

Alexander Pope

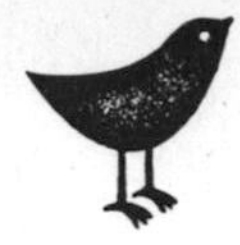

OH, TO BE 70 AGAIN.

Georges Clemenceau on his eightieth birthday

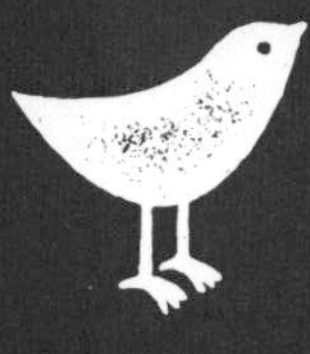

AGE, LIKE DISTANCE, LENDS A DOUBLE CHARM.

Oliver Wendell Holmes Jr

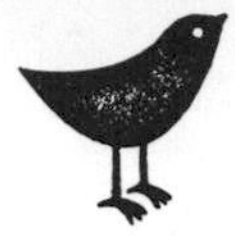

I HAVE ACHIEVED MY 70 YEARS IN THE USUAL WAY, BY STICKING STRICTLY TO A SCHEME OF LIFE WHICH WOULD KILL ANYBODY ELSE.

Mark Twain

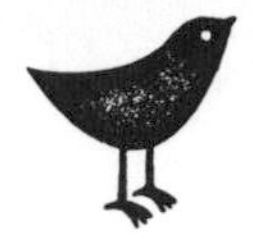

ON MY SEVENTIETH BIRTHDAY I FELT AS IF I WERE STANDING ON A MOUNTAIN HEIGHT... WHILE BEFORE ME, LIFE... SPREAD OUT GREEN, WILD, AND BEAUTIFUL.

Samuel Kirkland Lothrop

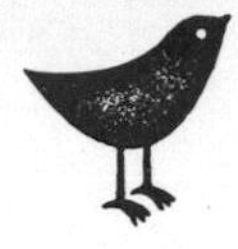

LET US CELEBRATE THE OCCASION WITH WINE AND SWEET WORDS.

Plautus

JUST WHAT I ALWAYS WANTED

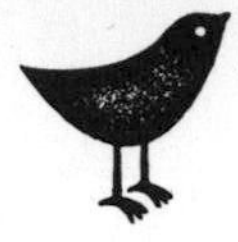

NOBODY CAN BE UNCHEERED WITH A BALLOON.

A. A. Milne

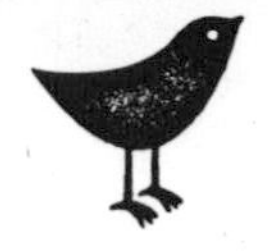

YESTERDAY IS HISTORY, TOMORROW IS A MYSTERY, BUT TODAY IS A GIFT. THAT IS WHY IT IS CALLED THE PRESENT.

Anonymous

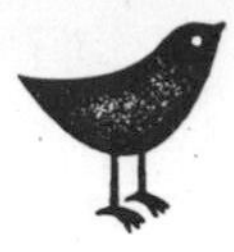

IF INSTEAD OF A GEM, OR EVEN A FLOWER, WE SHOULD CAST THE GIFT OF A LOVING THOUGHT INTO THE HEART OF A FRIEND, THAT WOULD BE GIVING AS THE ANGELS GIVE.

George MacDonald

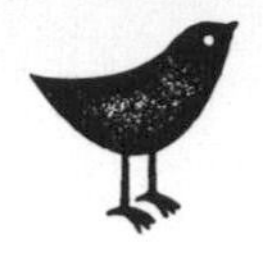

LIFE ISN'T TIED WITH A BOW BUT IT'S STILL A GIFT.

Anonymous

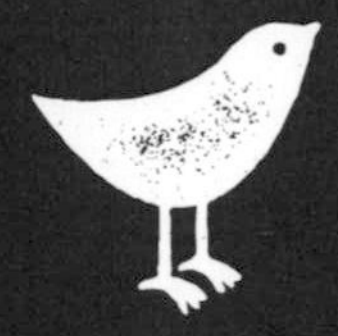

SURPRISE IS THE GREATEST GIFT WHICH LIFE CAN GRANT US.

Boris Pasternak

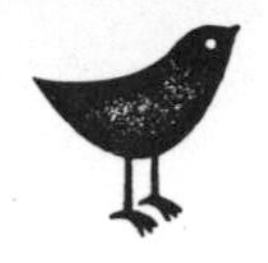

A GIFT, WITH A KIND COUNTENANCE, IS A DOUBLE PRESENT.

Proverb

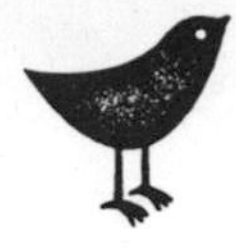

A GIFT CONSISTS NOT IN WHAT IS DONE OR GIVEN, BUT IN THE INTENTION OF THE GIVER OR DOER.

Seneca the Younger

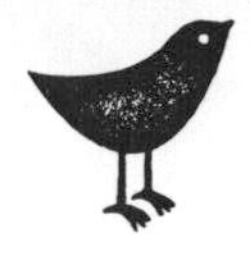

THE MORE CANDLES YOU
HAVE ON YOUR CAKE,
THE BIGGER THE WISH
YOU CAN MAKE.

Anonymous

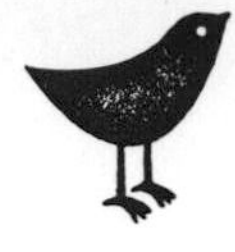

EACH DAY COMES
BEARING ITS OWN GIFTS.
UNTIE THE RIBBONS.

Ruth Ann Schabacker

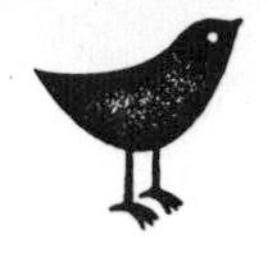

WHY IS A BIRTHDAY CAKE THE ONLY FOOD YOU CAN BLOW ON AND SPIT ON AND EVERYBODY RUSHES TO GET A PIECE?

Bobby Kelton

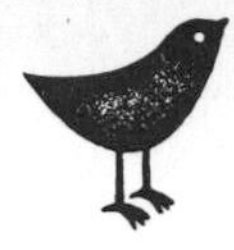

A HUG IS THE PERFECT GIFT; ONE SIZE FITS ALL, AND NOBODY MINDS IF YOU EXCHANGE IT.

Anonymous

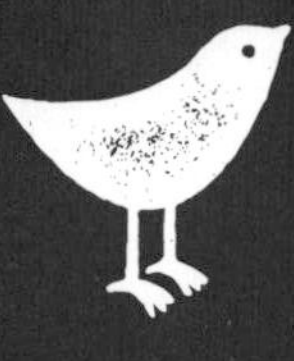

A COMFORTABLE OLD AGE IS THE REWARD OF A WELL-SPENT YOUTH.

Maurice Chevalier

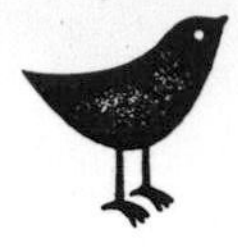

THE ABILITY TO LAUGH, ESPECIALLY AT OURSELVES, KEEPS THE HEART LIGHT AND THE MIND YOUNG.

Anonymous

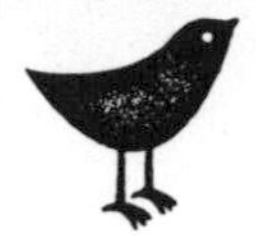

THERE ARE 364 DAYS WHEN YOU MIGHT GET UN-BIRTHDAY PRESENTS... AND ONLY ONE FOR BIRTHDAY PRESENTS, YOU KNOW.

Lewis Carroll

GRIN AND BEAR IT

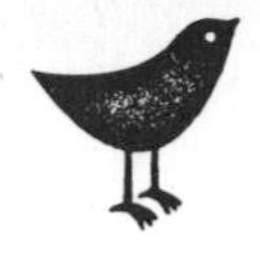

I WILL NEVER GIVE IN TO OLD AGE UNTIL I BECOME OLD. AND I'M NOT OLD YET!

Tina Turner

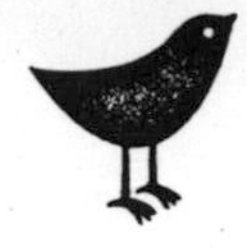

I STILL HAVE A FULL DECK; I JUST SHUFFLE SLOWER NOW.

Anonymous

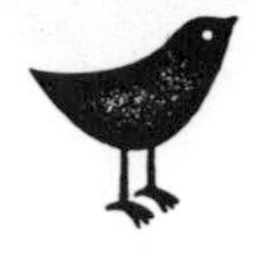

‘AGE’ IS THE ACCEPTANCE OF A TERM OF YEARS. BUT MATURITY IS THE GLORY OF YEARS.

Martha Graham

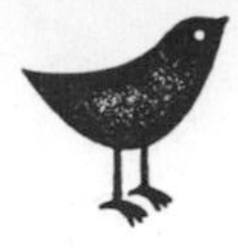

WE GROW NEITHER BETTER NOR WORSE AS WE GET OLD, BUT MORE LIKE OURSELVES.

May Lamberton Becker

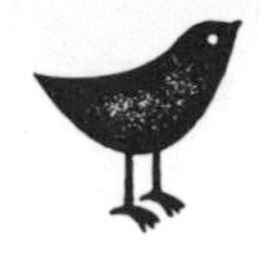

IT'S TIME TO START LIVING THE LIFE YOU'VE IMAGINED.

Henry James

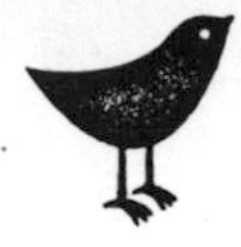

THE GREAT THING ABOUT GETTING OLDER IS THAT YOU DON'T LOSE ALL THE OTHER AGES YOU'VE BEEN.

Madeleine L'Engle

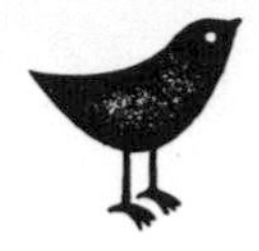

ONE OF THE ADVANTAGES OF BEING 70 IS THAT YOU ONLY NEED FOUR HOURS' SLEEP. TRUE, YOU NEED IT FOUR TIMES A DAY, BUT STILL.

Denis Norden

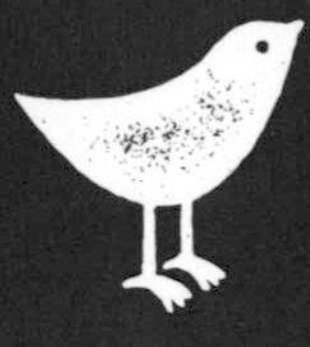

FATHER TIME IS NOT ALWAYS A HARD PARENT.

Charles Dickens

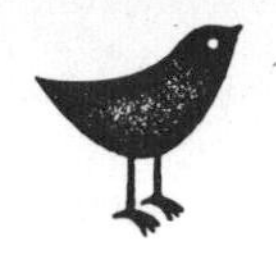

AGE IS A MATTER OF FEELING, NOT OF YEARS.

George William Curtis

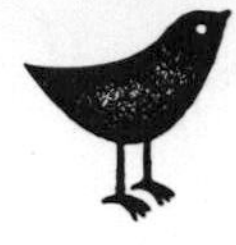

NO ONE IS SO OLD AS TO THINK HE CANNOT LIVE ONE MORE YEAR.

Cicero

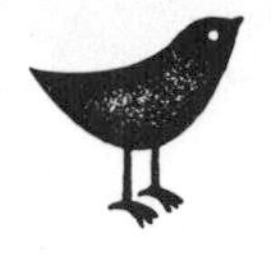

I AM GETTING TO AN AGE WHEN I CAN ONLY ENJOY THE LAST SPORT LEFT. IT IS CALLED HUNTING FOR YOUR SPECTACLES.

Edward Grey

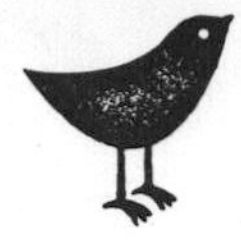

STOP WORRYING ABOUT THE POTHOLES IN THE ROAD AND CELEBRATE THE JOURNEY!

Anonymous

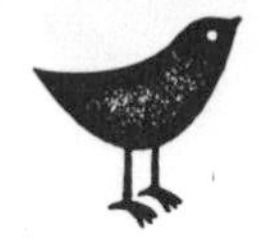

OLD AGE IS AN EXCELLENT TIME FOR OUTRAGE. MY GOAL IS TO SAY OR DO AT LEAST ONE OUTRAGEOUS THING EVERY WEEK.

Maggie Kuhn

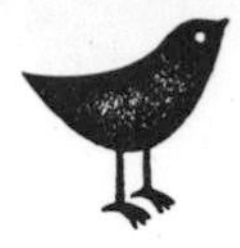

THE GREAT SECRET THAT ALL OLD PEOPLE SHARE IS THAT YOU REALLY HAVEN'T CHANGED... YOUR BODY CHANGES, BUT YOU DON'T CHANGE AT ALL.

Doris Lessing

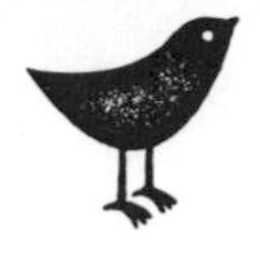

PERHAPS ONE HAS TO BE VERY OLD BEFORE ONE LEARNS TO BE AMUSED RATHER THAN SHOCKED.

Pearl S. Buck

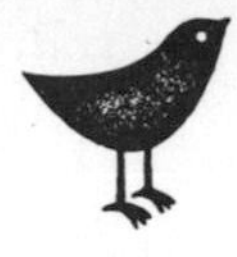

IF YOU SURVIVE LONG ENOUGH, YOU'RE REVERED – RATHER LIKE AN OLD BUILDING.

Katharine Hepburn

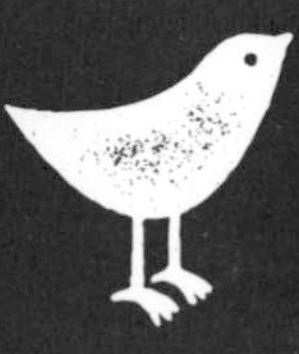

I'M GROWING OLD; I DELIGHT IN THE PAST.

Henri Matisse

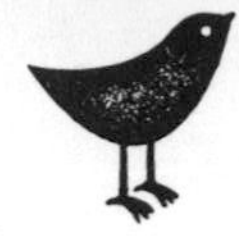

THE LONGER I LIVE
THE MORE BEAUTIFUL
LIFE BECOMES.

Frank Lloyd Wright

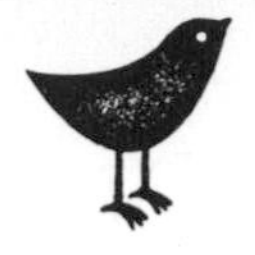

A HEALTHY OLD FELLOW,
THAT IS NOT A FOOL,
IS THE HAPPIEST
CREATURE LIVING.

Richard Steele

DO A
LITTLE
DANCE,
MAKE A
LITTLE
LOVE

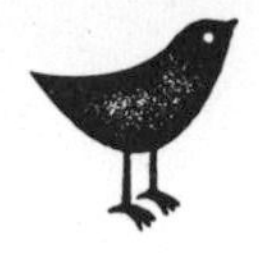

I CAN STILL ENJOY SEX AT 74. I LIVE AT 75, SO IT'S NO DISTANCE.

Bob Monkhouse

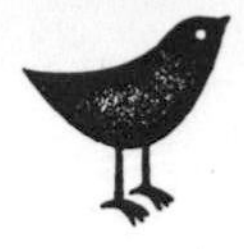

ONE OF THE BEST PARTS OF GROWING OLDER? YOU CAN FLIRT ALL YOU LIKE SINCE YOU'VE BECOME HARMLESS.

Liz Smith

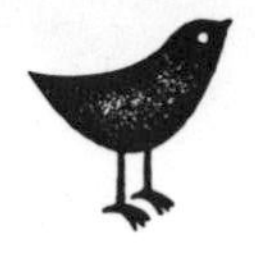

LAUGHTER DOESN'T REQUIRE TEETH.

Bill Newton

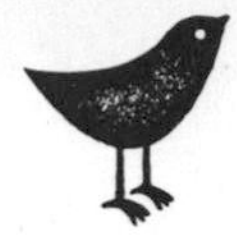

THE OTHER DAY A MAN ASKED ME WHAT I THOUGHT WAS THE BEST TIME OF LIFE. 'WHY,' I ANSWERED WITHOUT A THOUGHT, 'NOW.'

David Grayson

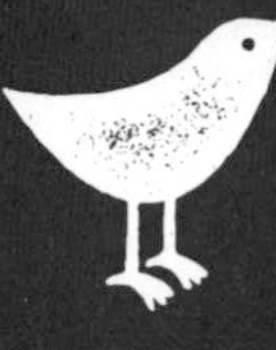

DON'T WAIT.
MAKE MEMORIES
TODAY.
CELEBRATE YOUR
LIFE!

Anonymous

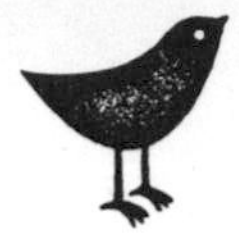

HER BIRTHDAY'S OUR
FETE DAY,
WE'LL MAKE IT OUR
GREAT DAY,
AND GIVE HER OUR
PRESENTS
AND SING HER OUR
SONG.

E. Nesbit

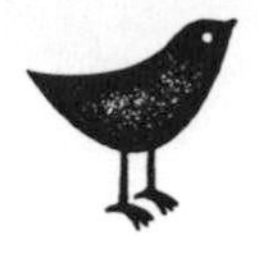

I CELEBRATE MYSELF, AND SING MYSELF.

Walt Whitman

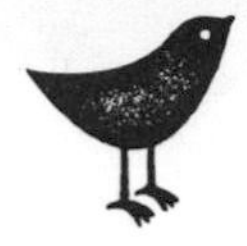

THE MORE YOU PRAISE AND CELEBRATE YOUR LIFE, THE MORE THERE IS IN LIFE TO CELEBRATE.

Oprah Winfrey

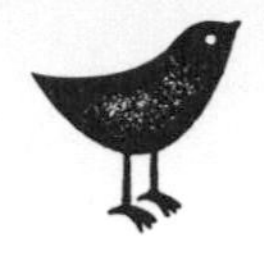

IT'S IMPORTANT TO HAVE A TWINKLE IN YOUR WRINKLE.

Anonymous

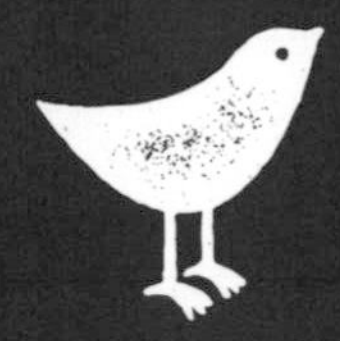

WITH MIRTH AND LAUGHTER LET OLD WRINKLES COME.

William Shakespeare

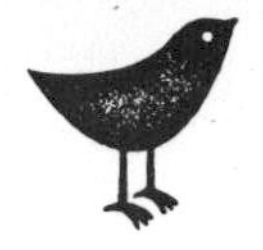

I ALWAYS MAKE A POINT OF STARTING THE DAY AT 6 A.M. WITH CHAMPAGNE. IT GOES STRAIGHT TO THE HEART AND CHEERS ONE UP.

John Mortimer

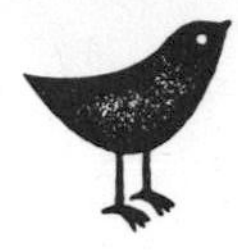

THE AGEING PROCESS HAS YOU FIRMLY IN ITS GRASP IF YOU NEVER GET THE URGE TO THROW A SNOWBALL.

Doug Larson

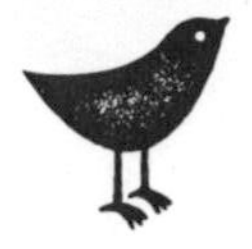

AS THIS AUSPICIOUS DAY BEGAN THE RACE OF EV'RY VIRTUE JOIN'D WITH EV'RY GRACE; MAY YOU, WHO OWN THEM, WELCOME ITS RETURN, TILL EXCELLENCE, LIKE YOURS, AGAIN IS BORN.

Lord Francis Jeffrey

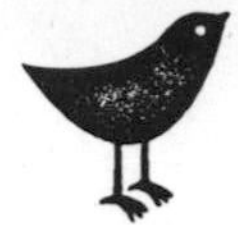

YOU ARE NEVER TOO OLD TO SET ANOTHER GOAL OR TO DREAM A NEW DREAM.

C. S. Lewis

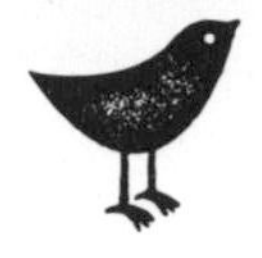

MY ADVICE FOR LIFE: DANCE AND SING YOUR SONG WHILE THE PARTY IS STILL ON.

Rasheed Ogunlaru

YOUNG AT HEART

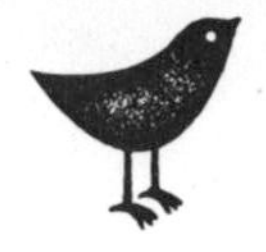

OLD AGE IS ALWAYS 15 YEARS OLDER THAN I AM.

Oliver Wendell Holmes Jr

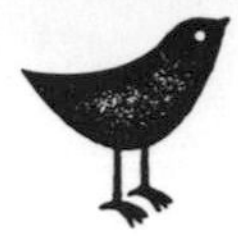

I'M SAVING THAT ROCKER FOR THE DAY WHEN I FEEL AS OLD AS I REALLY AM.

Dwight D. Eisenhower

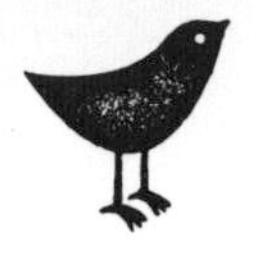

GRANDMAS ARE MUMS WITH LOTS OF FROSTING.

Anonymous

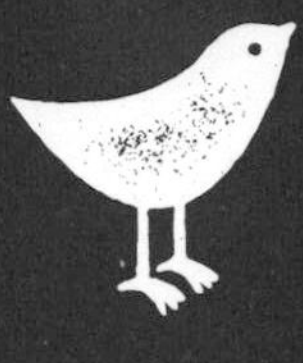

WE TURN NOT OLDER WITH YEARS, BUT NEWER EVERY DAY.

Emily Dickinson

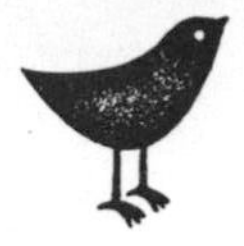

IN OUR DREAMS WE ARE ALWAYS YOUNG.

Sarah Louise Delany

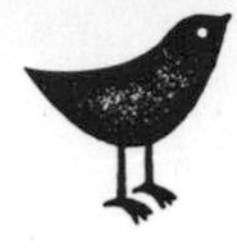

MAY YOU LIVE ALL THE DAYS OF YOUR LIFE.

Jonathan Swift

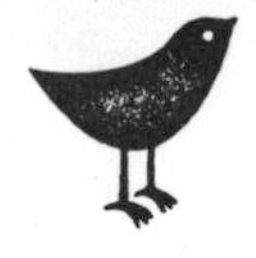

AGE IS JUST A NUMBER. IT'S TOTALLY IRRELEVANT UNLESS, OF COURSE, YOU HAPPEN TO BE A BOTTLE OF WINE.

Joan Collins

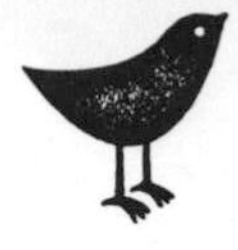

YOU'RE ONLY AS YOUNG AS THE LAST TIME YOU CHANGED YOUR MIND.

Timothy Leary

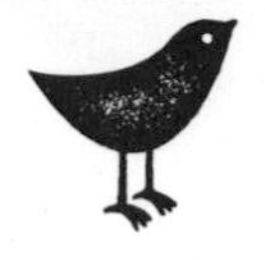

I'M HAPPY TO REPORT THAT MY INNER CHILD IS STILL AGELESS.

James Broughton

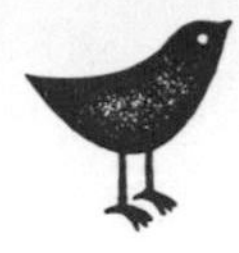

A WOMAN HAS THE RIGHT TO TREAT THE SUBJECT OF HER AGE WITH AMBIGUITY.

Helena Rubinstein

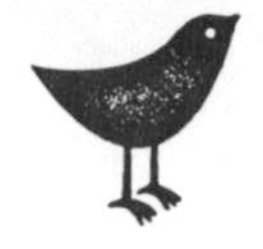

THERE ARE PEOPLE
WHOSE WATCH STOPS AT A
CERTAIN HOUR AND WHO
REMAIN PERMANENTLY
AT THAT AGE.

Charles Augustin Sainte-Beuve

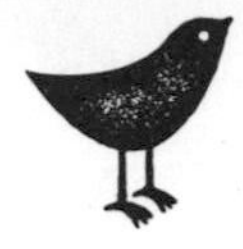

IN THE MIDST OF WINTER, I FINALLY LEARNED THAT THERE WAS IN ME AN INVINCIBLE SUMMER.

Albert Camus

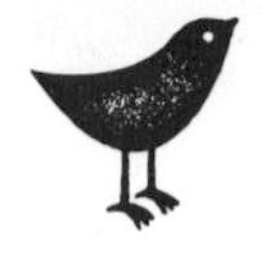

INSIDE EVERY OLDER PERSON IS A YOUNGER PERSON WONDERING WHAT THE HELL HAPPENED.

Cora Harvey Armstrong

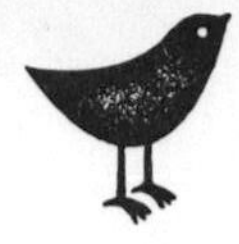

GETTING OLD AIN'T FOR SISSIES.

Bette Davis

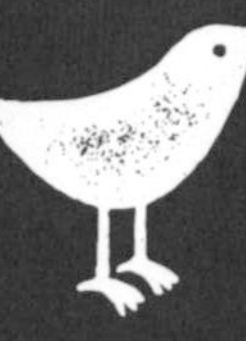

EVERYONE IS THE AGE OF THEIR HEART.

Guatemalan proverb

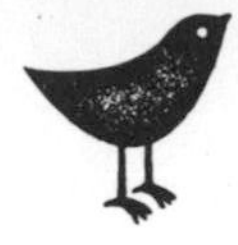

THE SECRET TO STAYING YOUNG IS TO LIVE HONESTLY, EAT SLOWLY, AND LIE ABOUT YOUR AGE.

Lucille Ball

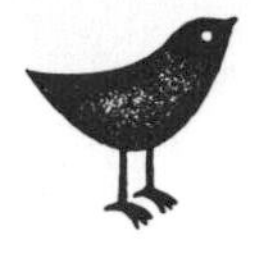

I'M NOT INTERESTED IN AGE. PEOPLE WHO TELL ME THEIR AGE ARE SILLY. YOU'RE AS OLD AS YOU FEEL.

Elizabeth Arden

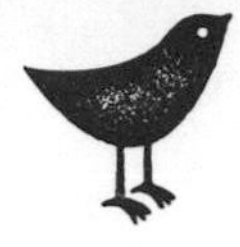

OLD AGE IS LIKE EVERYTHING ELSE. TO MAKE A SUCCESS OF IT, YOU'VE GOT TO START YOUNG.

Theodore Roosevelt

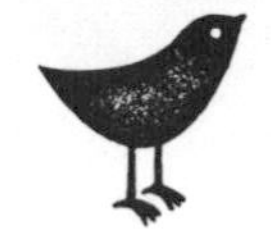

NATURE DOES NOT EQUALLY DISTRIBUTE ENERGY. SOME PEOPLE ARE BORN OLD AND TIRED WHILE OTHERS ARE GOING STRONG AT 70.

Dorothy Thompson

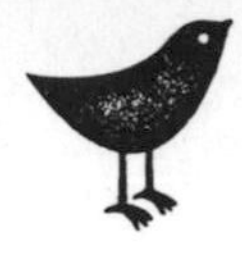

WHEN I WAS A BOY THE DEAD SEA WAS ONLY SICK.

George Burns

OLDER AND WISER?

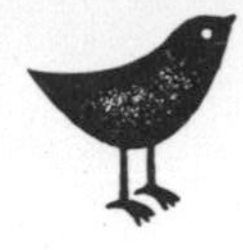

AS YOU GROW OLDER, YOU LEARN TO UNDERSTAND LIFE A LITTLE BETTER.

Solomon Burke

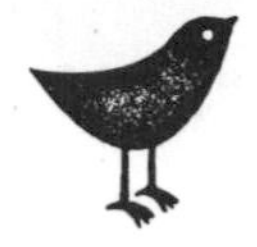

TO KEEP THE HEART UNWRINKLED, TO BE HOPEFUL, KINDLY, CHEERFUL, REVERENT – THAT IS TO TRIUMPH OVER OLD AGE.

Thomas Bailey Aldrich

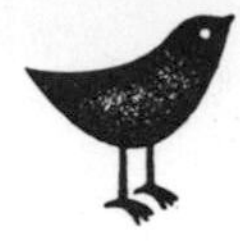

ALL LIFE IS AN EXPERIMENT. THE MORE EXPERIMENTS YOU MAKE THE BETTER.

Ralph Waldo Emerson

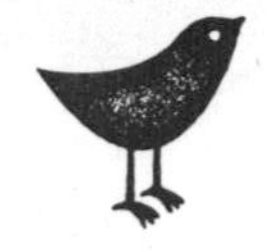

IF YOU CAN SPEND A PERFECTLY USELESS AFTERNOON IN A PERFECTLY USELESS MANNER, YOU HAVE LEARNED HOW TO LIVE.

Lin Yutang

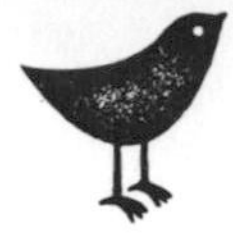

AS YOU GROW OLDER,
YOU WILL DISCOVER THAT
YOU HAVE TWO HANDS,
ONE FOR HELPING
YOURSELF, THE OTHER
FOR HELPING OTHERS.

Audrey Hepburn

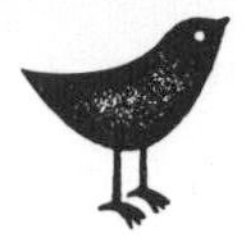

TO KNOW HOW TO GROW OLD IS THE MASTER WORK OF WISDOM, AND ONE OF THE MOST DIFFICULT CHAPTERS IN THE GREAT ART OF LIVING.

Henri-Frédéric Amiel

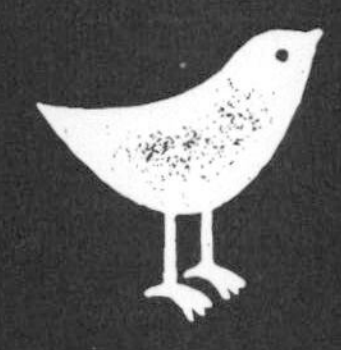

WE ARE NOT LIMITED BY OUR OLD AGE; WE ARE LIBERATED BY IT.

Stu Mittleman

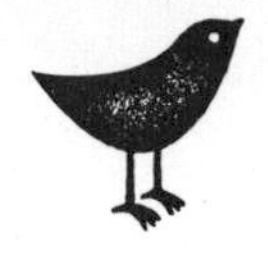

OLD AGE IS READY TO UNDERTAKE TASKS THAT YOUTH SHIRKED BECAUSE THEY WOULD TAKE TOO LONG.

W. Somerset Maugham

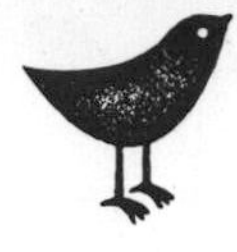

AGE IS AN
OPPORTUNITY
NO LESS THAN
YOUTH ITSELF.

Henry Wadsworth Longfellow

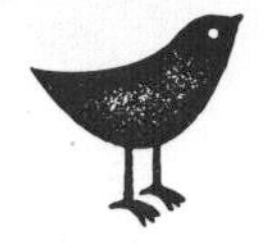

THE ELDERLY DON'T DRIVE THAT BADLY; THEY'RE JUST THE ONLY ONES WITH TIME TO DO THE SPEED LIMIT.

Jason Love

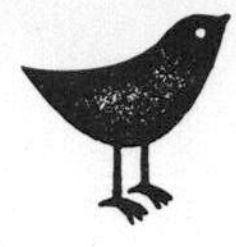

THEY TOLD ME IF I GOT OLDER I'D GET WISER. IN THAT CASE I MUST BE A GENIUS.

George Burns

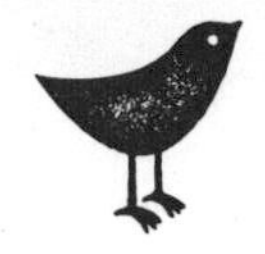

I'VE REACHED AN AGE WHEN I CAN'T USE MY YOUTH AS AN EXCUSE FOR MY IGNORANCE ANY MORE.

Helen-Janet Bonellie

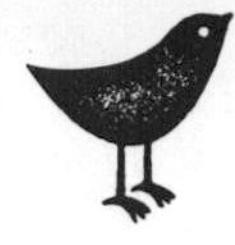

THE ONLY SOURCE OF KNOWLEDGE IS EXPERIENCE.

Albert Einstein

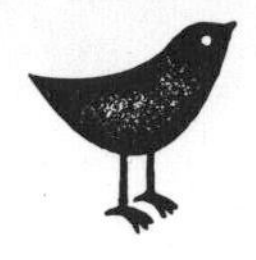

FEW PEOPLE KNOW HOW TO BE OLD.

François de La Rochefoucauld

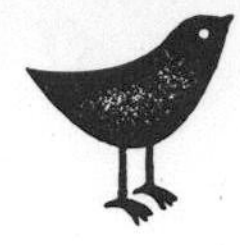

I LIKE BEST OF ALL AUTUMN, BECAUSE... ITS GOLDEN RICHNESS SPEAKS... OF THE MELLOWNESS AND KINDLY WISDOM OF APPROACHING AGE.

Lin Yutang

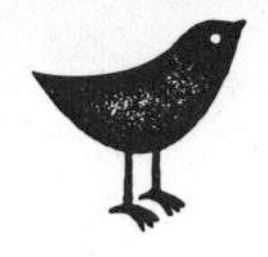

DON'T JUST COUNT YOUR YEARS, MAKE YOUR YEARS COUNT.

Ernest Myers

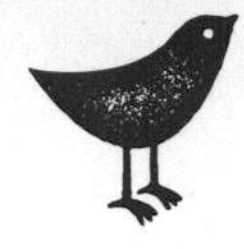

NO MAN IS EVER OLD ENOUGH TO KNOW BETTER.

Holbrook Jackson

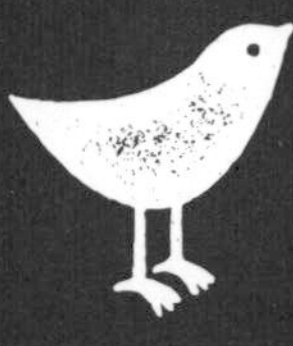

THE OLDER THE FIDDLE, THE SWEETER THE TUNE.

English proverb

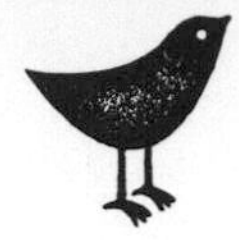

THE MORE SAND HAS ESCAPED FROM THE HOURGLASS OF OUR LIFE, THE CLEARER WE SHOULD SEE THROUGH IT.

Jean Paul

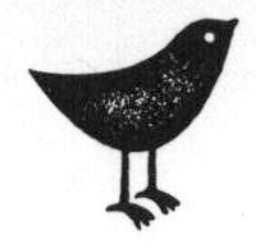

BORN TO BE WILD – LIVE TO OUTGROW IT.

Doug Horton

LIVE, LOVE AND LAST

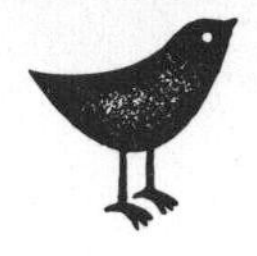

I'M TOO OLD TO DO THINGS BY HALF.

Lou Reed

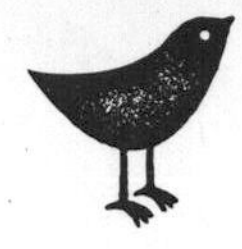

FEW THINGS ARE
MORE DELIGHTFUL
THAN GRANDCHILDREN
FIGHTING OVER
YOUR LAP.

Doug Larson

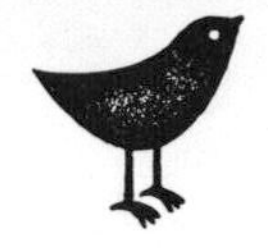

THE GOLDEN AGE
IS BEFORE US, NOT
BEHIND US.

Sallust

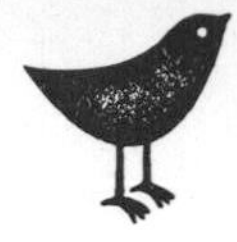

I LOVE EVERYTHING THAT'S OLD: OLD FRIENDS, OLD TIMES, OLD MANNERS, OLD BOOKS, OLD WINES.

Oliver Goldsmith

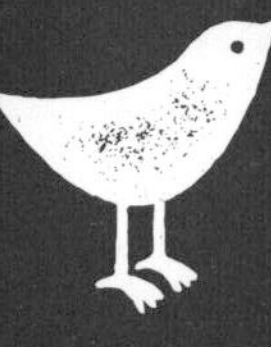

YOU ARE ONLY YOUNG ONCE, BUT YOU CAN BE IMMATURE FOR A LIFETIME.

John P. Grier

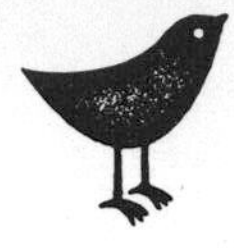

MY GRANDKIDS BELIEVE I'M THE OLDEST THING IN THE WORLD. AND AFTER TWO OR THREE HOURS WITH THEM, I BELIEVE IT, TOO.

Gene Perret

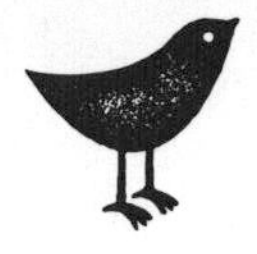

LIFE IS TOO SHORT, SO KISS SLOWLY, LAUGH INSANELY, LOVE TRULY AND FORGIVE QUICKLY.

Anonymous

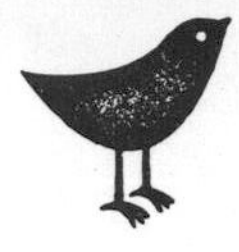

AT 70, I WOULD SAY THE ADVANTAGE IS THAT YOU TAKE LIFE MORE CALMLY. YOU KNOW THAT 'THIS, TOO, SHALL PASS!'

Eleanor Roosevelt

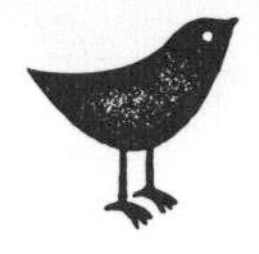

GOD GAVE US THE GIFT OF LIFE; IT IS UP TO US TO GIVE OURSELVES THE GIFT OF LIVING WELL.

Voltaire

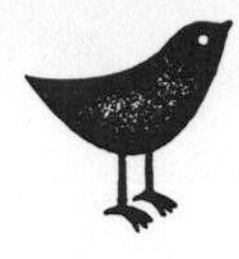

THE IMPORTANT THING IS NOT HOW MANY YEARS IN YOUR LIFE, BUT HOW MUCH LIFE IN YOUR YEARS!

Edward Stieglitz

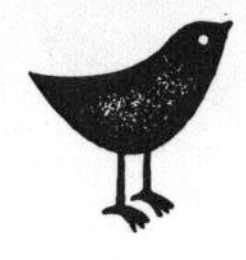

HE WHO LAUGHS, LASTS!

Mary Pettibone Poole

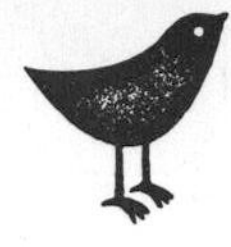

SO MAYST THOU LIVE,
DEAR! MANY YEARS,
IN ALL THE BLISS THAT
LIFE ENDEARS.

Thomas Hood

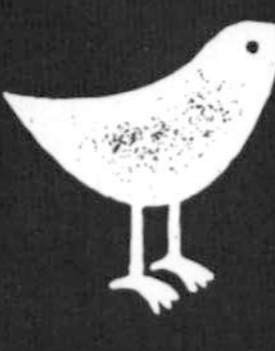

LIFE IS JUST ONE GRAND, SWEET SONG, SO START THE MUSIC.

Ronald Reagan

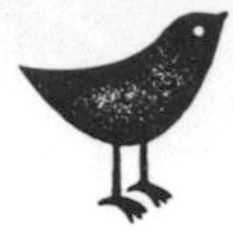

OLD AGE, BELIEVE ME, IS A GOOD AND PLEASANT THING. IT IS TRUE YOU ARE GENTLY SHOULDERED OFF THE STAGE, BUT THEN YOU ARE GIVEN SUCH A COMFORTABLE FRONT STALL AS SPECTATOR.

Jane Harrison

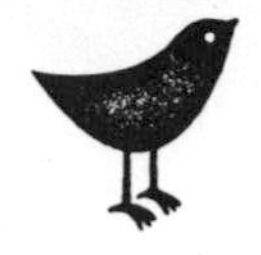

IF YOU ASSOCIATE
ENOUGH WITH OLDER
PEOPLE WHO ENJOY
THEIR LIVES, YOU WILL
GAIN THE POSSIBILITY
FOR A FULL LIFE.

Margaret Mead

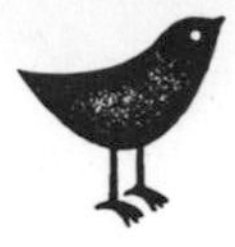

PEOPLE ARE ALWAYS ASKING ABOUT THE GOOD OLD DAYS. I SAY, WHY DON'T YOU SAY THE GOOD NOW DAYS?

Robert M. Young

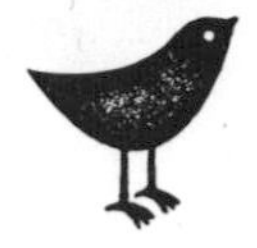

HERE, WITH WHITENED HAIR... HE DRANK TO LIFE, TO ALL IT HAD BEEN, TO WHAT IT WAS, TO WHAT IT WOULD BE.

Sean O'Casey

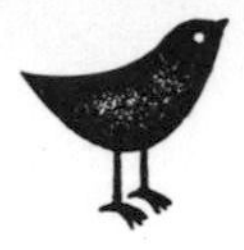

NO MATTER WHAT HAPPENS, I'M LOUD, NOISY, EARTHY AND READY FOR MUCH MORE LIVING.

Elizabeth Taylor

ILLS, PILLS AND TWINGES

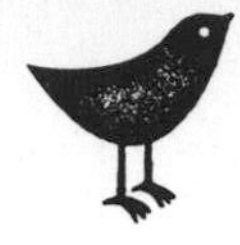

I DON'T DO ALCOHOL ANY MORE – I GET THE SAME EFFECT JUST STANDING UP FAST.

Anonymous

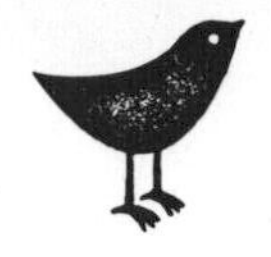

BEWARE OF THE YOUNG DOCTOR AND THE OLD BARBER.

Benjamin Franklin

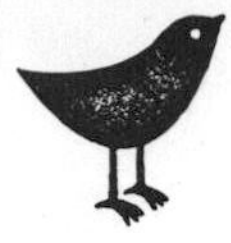

AS YOU GET OLDER THREE THINGS HAPPEN. THE FIRST IS YOUR MEMORY GOES, AND I CAN'T REMEMBER THE OTHER TWO...

Norman Wisdom

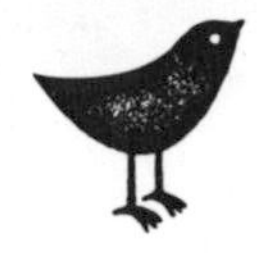

MY DOCTOR TOLD ME
TO DO SOMETHING
THAT PUTS ME OUT OF
BREATH, SO I'VE TAKEN
UP SMOKING AGAIN.

Jo Brand

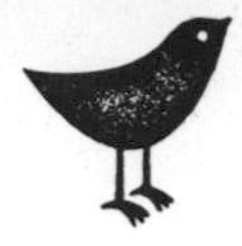

EVERYTHING SLOWS DOWN WITH AGE, EXCEPT THE TIME IT TAKES CAKE AND ICE CREAM TO REACH YOUR HIPS.

John Wagner

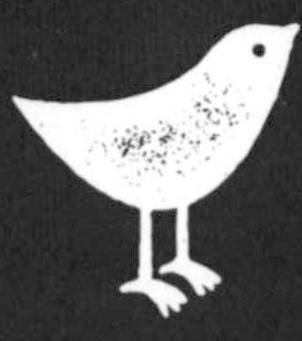

GRANT ME CHASTITY AND CONTINENCE, BUT NOT YET.

Augustine of Hippo

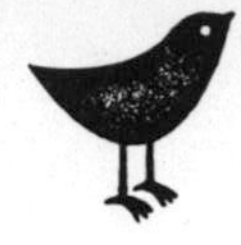

IF YOU REST,
YOU RUST.

Helen Hayes

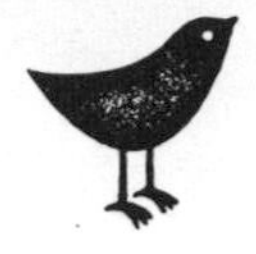

I'M AT AN AGE WHEN MY BACK GOES OUT MORE THAN I DO.

Phyllis Diller

CHIN UP, CHEST OUT

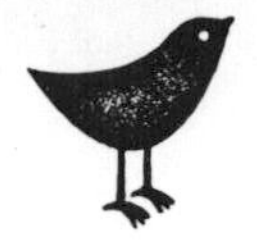

I DON'T GENERALLY FEEL ANYTHING UNTIL NOON, THEN IT'S TIME FOR MY NAP.

Bob Hope

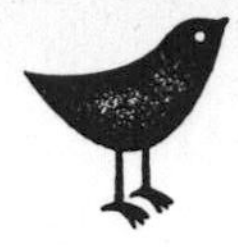

EVERY WRINKLE [IS] BUT A NOTCH IN THE QUIET CALENDAR OF A WELL-SPENT LIFE.

Charles Dickens

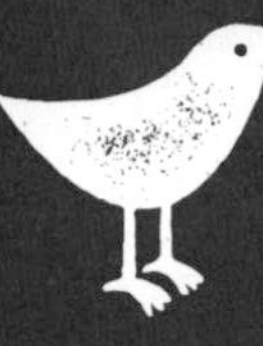

YOU CAN ONLY PERCEIVE REAL BEAUTY IN A PERSON AS THEY GET OLDER.

Anouk Aimée

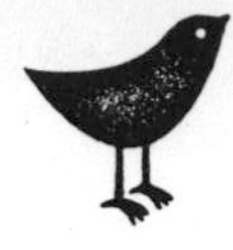

YOUTH IS THE GIFT OF NATURE, BUT AGE IS A WORK OF ART.

Garson Kanin

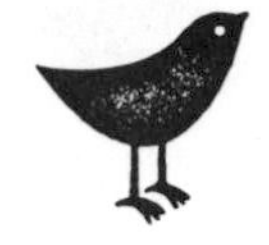

AGE SHOULD NOT HAVE ITS FACE LIFTED, BUT IT SHOULD RATHER TEACH THE WORLD TO ADMIRE WRINKLES AS THE ETCHINGS OF EXPERIENCE.

Ralph Barton Perry

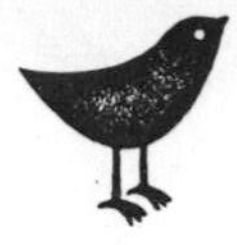

GOOD CHEEKBONES ARE THE BRASSIERE OF OLD AGE.

Barbara de Portago

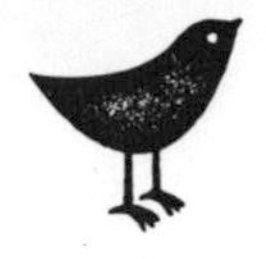

HOW PLEASANT IS THE DAY WHEN WE GIVE UP STRIVING TO BE YOUNG, – OR SLENDER.

William James

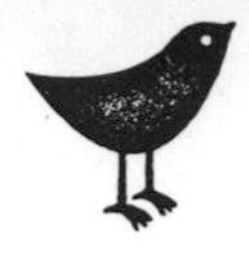

HOW BEAUTIFULLY LEAVES GROW OLD. HOW FULL OF LIGHT AND COLOUR ARE THEIR LAST DAYS.

John Burroughs

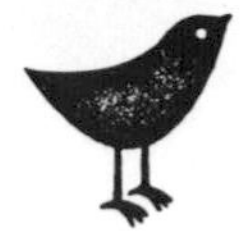

WHENEVER A MAN'S FRIENDS BEGIN TO COMPLIMENT HIM ABOUT LOOKING YOUNG, HE MAY BE SURE THAT THEY THINK HE IS GROWING OLD.

Washington Irving

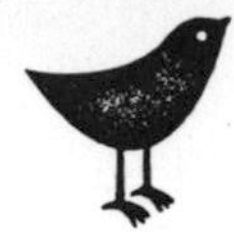

ANYONE WHO KEEPS THE ABILITY TO SEE BEAUTY NEVER GROWS OLD.

Franz Kafka

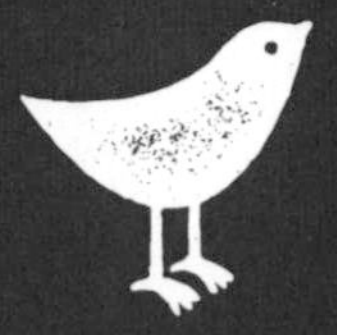

IT IS NOT HOW OLD YOU ARE, BUT HOW YOU ARE OLD.

Marie Dressler

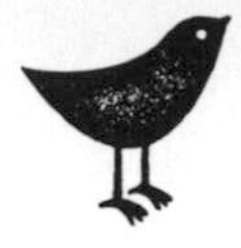

MIDDLE AGE IS WHEN YOUR BROAD MIND AND NARROW WAIST BEGIN TO CHANGE PLACES.

E. Joseph Cossman

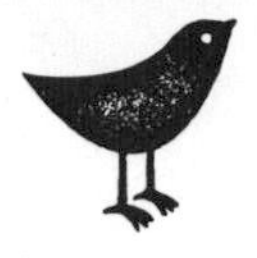

DON'T RETOUCH MY WRINKLES... I WOULD NOT WANT IT TO BE THOUGHT THAT I HAD LIVED FOR ALL THESE YEARS WITHOUT SOMETHING TO SHOW FOR IT.

Queen Elizabeth, The Queen Mother

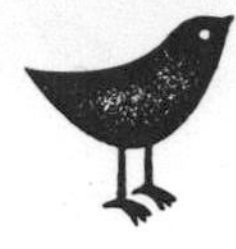

I'M LIKE OLD WINE. THEY DON'T BRING ME OUT VERY OFTEN, BUT I'M WELL PRESERVED.

Rose Fitzgerald Kennedy

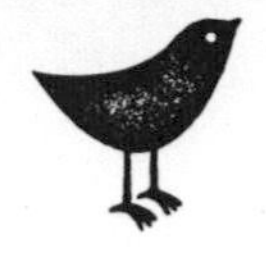

WRINKLES SHOULD MERELY INDICATE WHERE THE SMILES HAVE BEEN.

Mark Twain

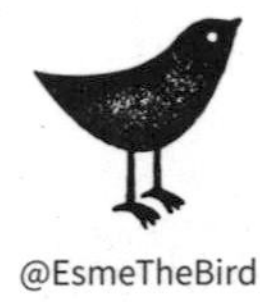

@EsmeTheBird

If you're interested in finding out more about our books, find us on Facebook at **Summersdale Publishers** and follow us on Twitter at **@Summersdale**.

www.summersdale.com